I0447746

FIBROMYALGIA - UNIFICATION THEORY; CONNECTING THE DOTS.

FIBROMYALGIA - UNIFICATION THEORY; CONNECTING THE DOTS.

Martin Morell MD

Copyright © 2017 Martin Morell MD
All rights reserved.

ISBN: 1540857638
ISBN 13: 9781540857637
Library of Congress Control Number: 2016920382
CreateSpace Independent Publishing Platform
North Charleston, South Carolina

Introduction

Just over a century ago schizophrenia was classified as a distinct mental disorder and originally divided into five types (DSM-III). Now genetic mapping has identified eight sub-types.[1]

Attention Deficit Hyperactivity Disorder was first described in the late 18th century.[2] Now we classify it by three distinct subtypes. For years, it was thought by many as the result of "bad parenting." Today we are learning about the role of molecular genetics and neuropsychological pathways, and sophisticated neuroimaging has further advanced our understanding of the condition.

Concepts of fibromyalgia may have dated back to Babylonian times.[3] For centuries, the disorder of global pain was known as muscular rheumatism. In 1904, Gowers coined the name fibrositis and not until 1972, did Smithe describe fibromyalgia (FM) as resulting in widespread pain and tender points. The first American College of Rheumatology criteria was published in 1990.[4] During that time, neurologists did not have a standardized neurological test; perhaps longstanding skepticism and constellation of co-morbid symptoms dissuaded many physicians from getting involved in treating it.

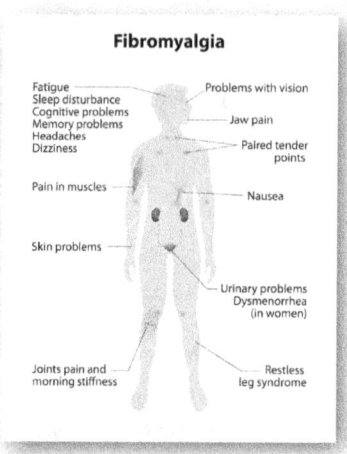

This book has been more than 10 years in the making. It incorporates reviews of worldwide literature on the subject and attempts to connect all the dots, from peripheral electrical signals that become amplified and the devastating downstream effect it has on global brain function. These brain functions influence not only neurotransmission, but also the neuroendocrine systems that contribute to such conditions as chronic fatigue and memory changes, among others.

"Differential Diagnosis"

As clinicians, we must make sure to exclude conditions that can mimic fibromyalgia.

1. Hypothyroidism
2. Severe vitamin D deficiency
3. Polymyalgia rheumatica (If over age 55)
4. Gluten sensitivity/allergy
5. Sleep apnea

6. Autoimmune conditions (i.e., lupus, rheumatoid arthritis)
7. Metastatic cancer
8. Cholesterol medications (highly lipophilic)
9. Depression
10. Myotonic dystrophy Type II

Fibromyalgia is a neurological disorder. Its epicenter is in sensory ascending fibers in the spinal cord. These nerve fibers have undergone biochemical changes, which cause amplified electrical waves that overtime have a devastating effect in various areas of brain function.

So why do most FM patients hurt when grabbed by the arm or when something is pressed against their skin? Normal pain conduction pathways (nociceptive) alert us when we face potential bodily harm. There are three steps in this process, involving thermal, mechanical or chemical signals that are converted to electrical signals. Like in an electrical appliance cord, the impulse travels across nerve synapses, activating upstream neurons in the spinal cord all the way to higher centers in the brain. Overtime, this impulse spreads out of control like a wild forest fire.

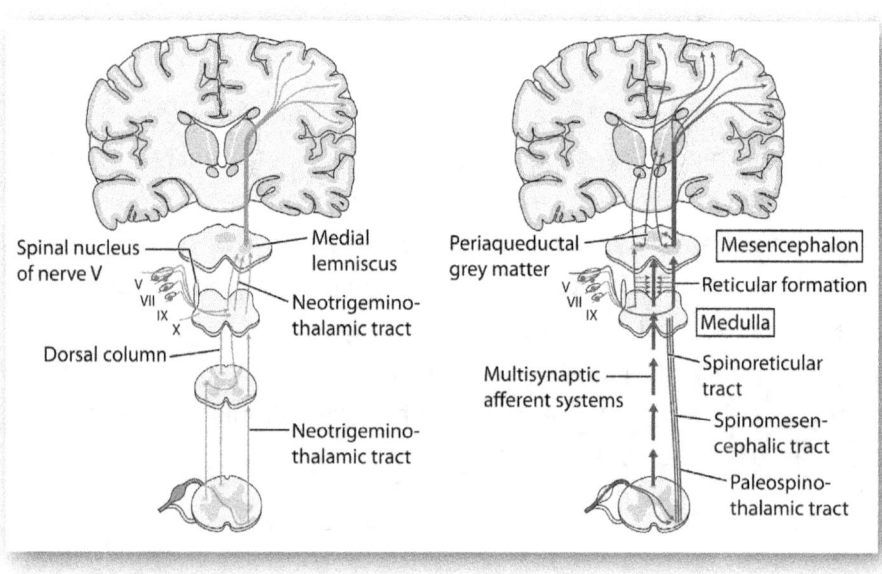

Spinal nucleus of nerve V

Medial lemniscus

Neotrigemino-thalamic tract

Dorsal column

Neotrigemino-thalamic tract

Periaqueductal grey matter

Mesencephalon

Reticular formation

Medulla

Multisynaptic afferent systems

Spinoreticular tract

Spinomesen-cephalic tract

Paleospino-thalamic tract

n the mammalian system, small unmyelinated "slow" conducting fibers respond to warmth while thinly myelinated A delta fibers (faster conduction) and C fibers respond to cold stimuli. (The type of fibers may explain why patients with FM respond differently to temperature variations). These receptors occupy most of the surface area, hence making trigger point identification obsolete.

These signals from activated pressure/temperature receptors converge near the spinal cord, entering it and crossing into the "posterolateral tract" through the dorsal root ganglion cells. These axons then enter either above or below nearby spinal segments before penetrating the grey matter in the dorsal horn. Here they synapse on second order neurons, continuing on the ipsilateral half of the spinal cord.

The electrical signals ascend the spinal cord, through the spinothalamic tract on the way to the thalamus in the brain. But the "highway" to the thalamus are several, some located posteriorly, laterally or even anteriorly on the outer spinal cord. (This could explain why spinal cord stimulators are not 100 percent efficient.)

The core problem in fibromyalgia centers in the spinothalamic tract, where the amplification of all incoming electrical signals create havoc (spinal or central sensitization) upstairs in the brain. Let us not forget that such sensitization can also occur peripherally, such as in the case with "shingles," or post herpetic neuralgia.

But the brain just does not sit there to take this abuse. Initially it attempts to extinguish such pain by feedback reflexes (successes occurring) in most acute pain events. However, with chronic stimuli, pain is experienced after peripheral receptors have been activated even if surrounding tissues have recovered.

It is possible that the descending pathways attempts to extinguish chronic pain are responsible for changes and sensitization of peripheral nociceptors[5]. Changes on peripheral Schwann cells in the skin of fibromyalgia patients have been described[6] and more recently, some have suggested an increase in sensory nerve fibers at specific sites in blood vessels in the skin.[7]

SPINAL CORD

There are three major sensory tracts:

- Posterior Column tract
- Spinothalamic tract
- Spinocerebellar tract

Each tract is further subdivided in two tracts, conveying information about light touch, pressure and temperature sensations. Additionally, there are other tracts like spino-olivary fibers.

At the molecular level, we have a large group of neurotransmitter and receptors that work to amplify the electrical signals traveling from first order neurons to second order neurons.

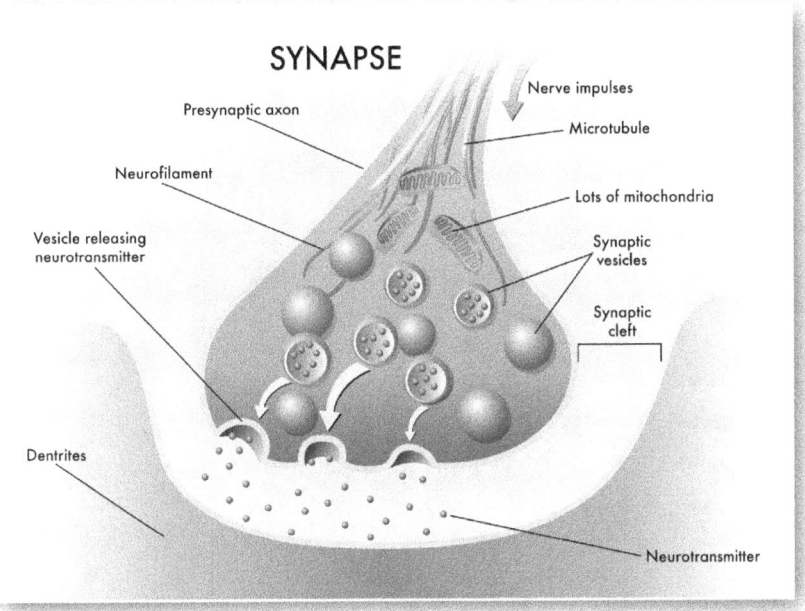

Among them are

Excitatory amino acids

- L Glutamate
- L Aspartate

Receptors

- NMDA (types 1 and 2)
- Kiamic acid (KA) receptors (high and low affinity)
- AMPA receptors
- Group I metabotropic receptors: mGluRI, mGluRs
- Group II metabotropic receptors: mGluR2-4 and 6

Inhibitory amino acids

- GABA
- glycine

Peptides

- Substance P
- Neurokinin A
- Calcitonin gene-related peptide
- Opioid peptides, encephalins and dymorphins
- Nociceptors
- Nocistatin

Biogenic amines

- Serotonin (5-HT)
- Norepinephrine (NE)
- Dopamine (DA)
- Acetylcholine (Ach)

ATP and adenosine receptors
Nitric oxide
Capsaicin and vanilloid receptors

- Histamine
- Prostaglandin
- Bradykinin
- Nerve growth factor

We only have but a few drugs that may block the action of these neurotransmitters on their receptor. There currently isn't a cure for FM, just treatment that may ameliorate the pain in some patients.

Spinal cord stimulators cost more than $50,000, helping some patients to a certain degree. Unfortunately, they do not reach deep, anterior pathways of the spinothalamic tract. It is possible that Nano-technology could be applied in the future.

BRAIN EVENTS

Numerous morphologic and biochemical events occur from the relentless augmented pain signals that enter deeper structures of the brain.[8]

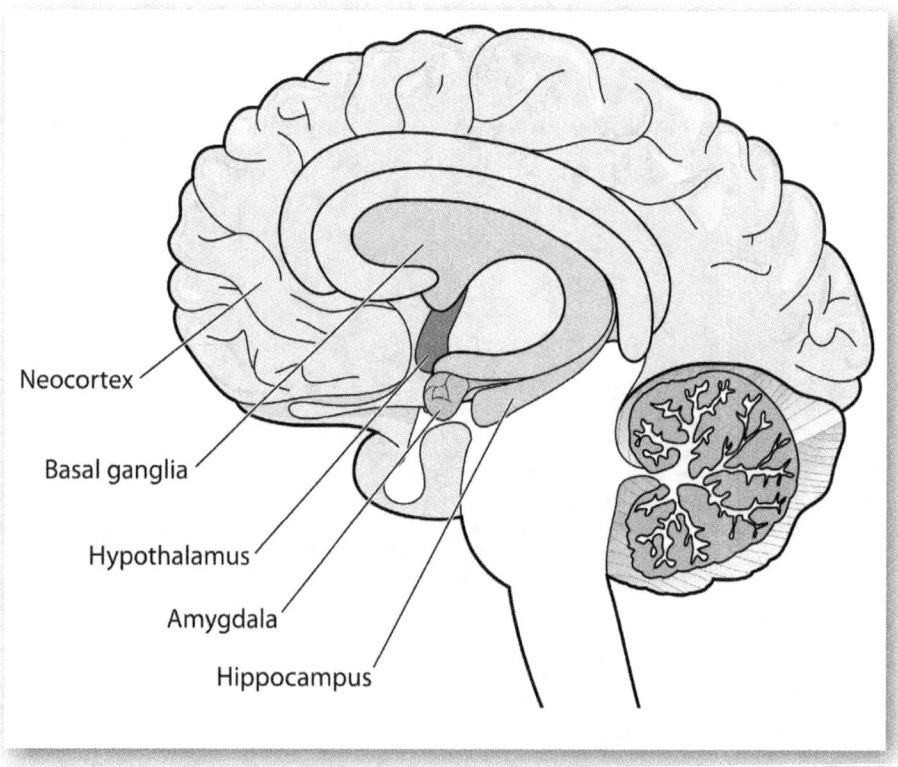

Neocortex

Basal ganglia

Hypothalamus

Amygdala

Hippocampus

So far, we have suggested that pain signal augmentation in the spinal cord is the epicenter of fibromyalgia. These signals are constantly traveling upward once any sensory receptor is activated peripherally such as a person grabbing the patient's limb. Even moving about in bed can result in pain for an individual with FM.

These bundles of nerve fibers then pass through the brainstem structures (Medulla Oblongata, Pons) into the hypothalamus. Now, guess what the hypothalamus does for a living?

1) Temperature regulation (shivering)
2) Endocrine control/ gonadotropic (involved in sex differentiation in the embryo)
3) Emotional reaction
4) Sleep and wakefulness/circadian (suprachiasmatic)
5) Stress control
6) Thirst and autonomic control (blood pressure, heart rate)
7) Short-term memory (mammillary bodies)

Think of what happens when you get electrical surges and how they interact with your household appliances. Many would be affected unless you have a surge protector: a hint to future possible therapies. Before we go into a bit more detail in what happens in these areas of the brain, let's look at some of the symptoms patients with FM describe and compare them to the list above.

1) Cold or heat intolerance
2) Pituitary – adrenal axis variations (As cluster, see ref.)
3) Depression/irritability
4) Fatigue/disrupted sleep
5) Anxiety
6) Irritable bowel
7) Paresthesia's, extremity numbness

We frequently hear how perception of heat and cold varies significantly in patients with FM. The spectrum is varied, as some people prefer warmer or colder environments to find "relief." (Some would prefer a warm Jacuzzi, while others cannot stand the heat.) The hypothalamus is an important homeostatic center for temperature control.

Regarding endocrine variations, the hypothalamic links the nervous system to the endocrine system via the pituitary gland. The hypothalamus does stimulate or inhibit pituitary hormones. Patients with FM exhibit a hypoactive sympatho-adrenal system as compared to controls during static exercise.[9] There are also decreased levels of prolactin and growth hormone in these individuals.[10]

The dorsomedial thalamus encodes emotional aspects of pain, so biochemical changes here may explain observed symptoms in patients with FM.

SLEEP DISTURBANCES

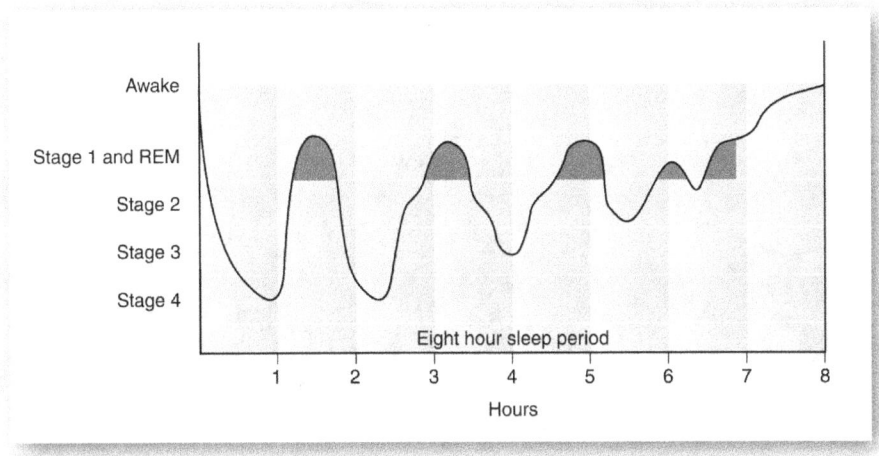

Studies comparing FM vs. non-FM patients during stage 4 sleep deprivation showed that both groups exhibited anomalous alpha rhythms in non-rapid eye movement (NREM) sleep EEG. This alpha-delta sleep contributes to the appearance of unwanted temporary musculoskeletal and mood symptoms in controls.

These deep stages of sleep are interrupted in patients with FM. This may explain the lack of dreaming in many patients with FM during REM sleep.

WAKEFULNESS AND FATIGUE

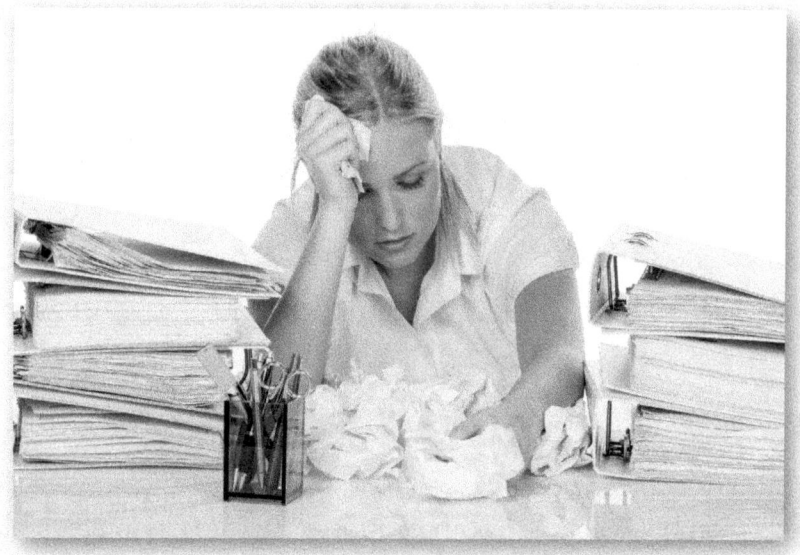

As higher mammals, we have developed two main areas that control wakefulness, the reticulate activating system (RAS) located in the midbrain and rich in dopamine tract projecting into the cerebral cortex, and the hypothalamic-mediated wakefulness rich in histamine-3- production (histamine 1 is associated with mechanism of itch in the skin), and histamine -2 with acid production on the gastrointestinal tracts.

In the hypothalamus, there are many nuclei with distinct functions. Of these, the "wake- promoting" tuberomammillary nuclei (TMN); the "trigger" suprachiasmatic nuclei; and the "sleep nuclei," the ventrolateral pre-optic area, play a significant role in wakefulness, attention and sleep.

Chronically augmented signals arriving from the spinothalamic tracts in FM disrupt the natural functioning balance in these areas. They adversely affect sleep[11], concentration and wakefulness. We do have medications that will enhance these functions by antagonizing histamine-3 reuptake and by inhibiting orexin thereby promoting sleep. (Refer to treatment of FM section.)

ANXIETY AND STRESS

There are many factors that contribute to anxiety and stress, such as chronic child/spousal abuse, sleep deprivation, anorexia nervosa and PTSD to mention a few. Like FM, these conditions contribute to atrophy in some areas in the brain. The constant influx of augmented pain signals in FM cause prolonged stress that increase glucocorticoid (stress hormone) levels by the hypothalamic-pituitary—adrenal (HPA) axis. This leads to increased glutaminergic signals, dendritic nerve remodeling and impaired neurogenesis.[12]

Besides the mammillary bodies in the hypothalamic, the hippocampus is involved in short-term memory, sleep regulation and nociceptive (pain) experience. Stress situations increase stress hormone levels that augment hippocampal NMDA (glutamate receptors) activity.[13] Glutamate is a major excitatory neurotransmitter in pain pathways and utilizes sodium channel receptors that promote neuronal depolarization.

Short-term memory is frequently affected in patients with FM due to hippocampal dysfunction.[14]

Chronic stress will also lead to atrophy in other important brain areas like the insula, which plays a role in speech. (Patients with FM frequently have difficulty putting sentences together.) The insula also affects taste, auditory systems and somatosensory and visceral (gut) pain processing.

Chronic pain also can result in atrophy and shrinkage of the prefrontal cortex and thalamus by as much as 11 percent in size![15] This contributes to decreased attention span and concentration ability, a common finding in FM patients. The atrophy that develops may be explained by hormonal, immune dysfunction, increase cortisol levels and blood flow alterations[16].

The thalamus-named subdivisions connect with the prefrontal cortex, insula and other brain areas that link to the somatosensory cortex. (Lesions of stroke victims reflect in the contralateral body site specific to the body region.) Perhaps these variations in activity and dynamic events explain numbness in the extremities experienced in FM. The thalamic signaling to the prefrontal cortex also contain the emotional aspect of pain, its intensity and project temperature and pressure information to the primary somatosensory cortex.

PARESTHESIA'S AND NUMBNESS OF EXTREMITIES IN FM

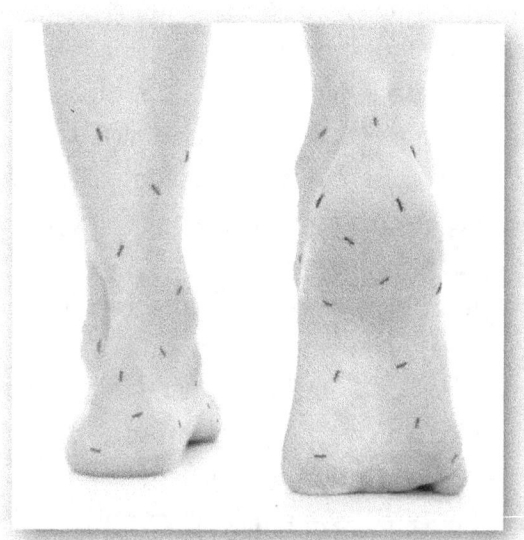

Patients with FM frequently complain of numbness in one or several extremities. Many undergo nerve conduction test that often fails to identify a cause. As suggested earlier, we propose that alterations in upstream nerve conduction and signal amplification, global atrophy in specific brain areas and variation in neurochemistry and brain wave activity affect the sensory perception at the cortical homunculus (primary somatosensory cortex). Thalamic stroke victims have a similar experience, perceiving pain and/or burning in contralateral extremities.

IRRITABLE BOWEL

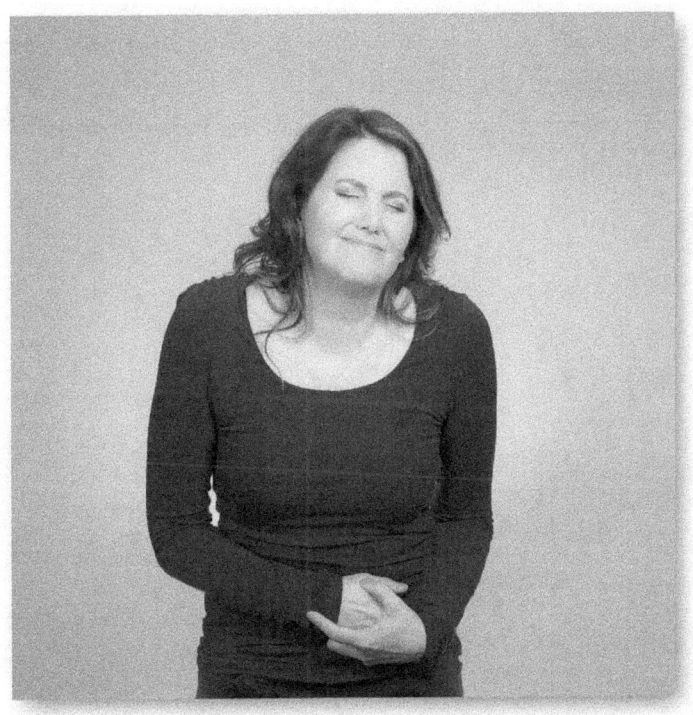

Did you know that most serotonin (5HT) is not in the brain but in the gastric tract? When people say, "I have a gut feeling," that is the serotonin talking! Ninety-five percent of serotonin is in the gut. Its levels increase in individuals with diarrhea and Celiac disease and decrease with constipation.[17] High concentrations of 5HT are released by the lamina propria: the neurotransmitter is absorbed by nerve terminals in enterocytes and vascular endothelial cell by co-active transport with Na+ and serotonin transporter (SERT). This SERT presence is higher in the small intestine than in other areas in the gut. In the future, more effective drugs will target type 1 tryptophan hydroxylase-1, the rate limiting enzyme for 5-HT synthesis.[18] Currently there are several 5-HT subtypes (1-5) agonist and antagonist in development.

Let us not forget, that in FM, HP axis activation produces increased cortisol levels, which affects irritable bowel syndrome, depression, anxiety and other functions. Increased urinary catecholamine's and cortisol have been measured in women with irritable bowel syndrome.[19]

SHORT-TERM MEMORY AND DECREASED CONCENTRATION

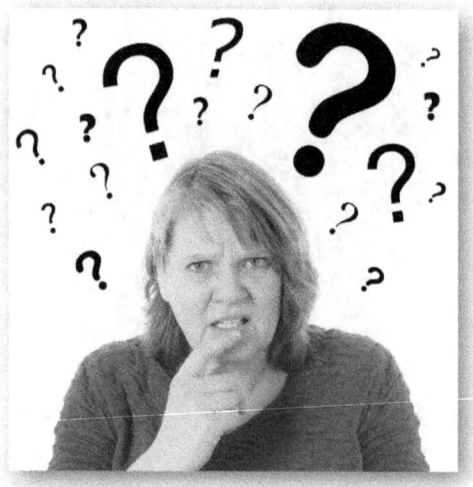

We mentioned earlier that constant stress/pain causes hippocampus dysfunction and shrinkage in an area key to short-term memory. Mammillary areas in the hypothalamus that play a role in memory are also affected. Additionally, EEG studies have shown dysfunction of sleep brain wave frequency. However, such findings also have been observed in diurnal (wake) measurements of superficial brain wave activity![20] Our multidisciplinary group could collect preliminary data on a brain wave alteration comparison between FM patients and controls through superficial EEG recording while doing a "stressful" brain activity: mathematical regression. The controls exhibited normal, fast B brain wave activity, while FM patients showed variation in brain waves (alpha and theta intrusions). It's possible these brain wave intrusions affect the ability of patients with FM to concentrate as well as their short-term memory.

Bandwidth	Frequency	
Delta:	0- 3.5 Hz	Pre-Sleep
Theta:	35-74 Hz	
Alpha:	74-12.1 Hz	
Beta:	12.1-40 Hz	Fully Awake

DEPRESSION AND COMORBIDITIES /DEPRESSION AND FM

In the "old" days, people believed FM syndrome was caused by depression. In fact, the similarities of metabolic and volumetric changes[21] are quite-eye opening. Similar structures shrink or atrophy sometimes 5-11 percent! Areas include both diseases:

- Prefrontal cortex (rich in Dopa and Serotonin)
- Insula (affective dimension of pain)
- Amygdala (aroma, music processing)

- Hippocampus (learning, memory, HPA regulator)
- Nucleus accumbens (reward, laugh, pleasure, addiction)

Newer technology and imaging studies have shed light on these mechanisms. They include:

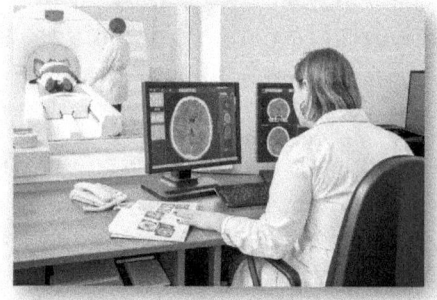

- Functional MRI
- Single Photon CT
- PET
- MR Spectroscopy (diffu-sion-weighted imaging & diffusion tension)[22]

Similarities of endocrine and neurochemical changes between FM and MDD include:

- Initial increase in activity HPA (hypothalamic-pituitary –adrenal axis, causing increase adrenal cortisol and catecholamine's.
- Increase cortisol leads to altered glycemic and lipid control (pro-inflammatory)
- Sleep disruption (due to alpha and other wave intrusion)
- Hormonal changes (including growth hormone and cortisol)
- Macrophage release of TNF and 11-6 (pro-inflammatory cytokines)
- Decreased levels of brain-derived nerve growth factors (BDNGF)
- Decreases in Substance P receptor expression (anti-depres-sant increase BDNGF)
- Increases in neurokinin at hippocampus (excitatory peptide)

DESCENDING PAIN SUPPRESSION SYSTEMS

Activation of mesolimbic dopamine neurons work well in acute pain. In chronic pain situations, this dopamine secretion decreases substantially at the nucleus accumbens, with further downstream decreases of endogenous opioids and increases in Substance P.

Similarly, these descending inhibitory systems involve serotonin and noradrenergic pathways. These have been measured in cerebrospinal fluids of patients.[23]

Some of the new drugs approved by the FDA appear to work in these areas.

Opioid receptors are also impaired in FM, as measured by positron emission tomography scanning (R. Harris, PhD, Department of Anesthesiology and Research, University of Michigan, Ann Arbor).

Studies in mice further shed light into the role of transcription inhibition of the prodynorphin (PRODINORPAIN) gene. The binding of a calcium-regulated transcription factor to downstream regulatory element regulator (DREAM) affects nociceptive transmission.[24]

So, thus far, we see how midbrain structural alterations from constant nociception may affect descending function of suppression systems. We postulate these defective systems contribute to electron-microscopic evidence of unmyelinated Schwann nerve fibers as described by the Koreans.[5]

GENETICS

Our clinic has seen 4,000 patients with FM over the past 12 years. Others have described subgroups of FM. The biggest group observed seem to have suffered injuries to the cervical or lumbar spine, such as whiplash or certain medical procedures resulting in pain that does not extinguish. Once again, like the earlier wild fire analogy, the pain burns out of control and expands in areas above and below the site of injury, becoming wide spread.

A second identifiable group in our studies includes those who have experienced adverse childhood trauma (Dr. J. Joseph) such as physical or emotional abuse. A third group involves flu-like symptoms that do not resolve. Psychological factors add to this complex picture.[25]

Are genetic factors involved? The answer could lie in the GCHI gene, a key modulator of pain sensitivity.[26] The enzyme produced by this gene interacts with various regulatory molecules involved in 6-protein coupled receptors (GPCR) signaling. (Editorial: Orin & Ablin, Clinical Highlights from the Rheumatologist, March 2013, volume 2, issue 3.)

The peptide produced by the GCHI gene serves as catalytic rate limiting step to produce (BH-4) tetrahydrobiopterin. BH-4 is a cofactor of many pain modulatory mediators, including nitrous oxide (NO) production. Preliminary evidence suggests human chromosome #17.

Furthermore, recent evidence suggests aggregates in families[27] in three candidate genes that play a role in pain modulation (TAAR1, R654 & CNR1).

Excluding parent modeling or conversion disorders, publications describe the incidence, age of onset and differential diagnosis of children with Juvenile Primary Fibromyalgia Syndrome.[28]

Other studies have demonstrated that adult patients who suffered childhood trauma exhibit decrease or flattened diurnal cortisol levels from collected saliva samples.[29]

FIBROMYALGIA TREATMENT

There are a high number of neurotransmitters and molecules that contribute to pain amplification in spinal pathways. To date, there are only a few FDA-approved treatments available, but these helps more than a third of patients that try them. Drug sensitivity, side effects or lack of efficacy account for most of the failures.

To simplify treatment for fibromyalgia, we've broken it down into three categories:

- Sleep
- Daytime pain control
- Energy and concentration

Sleep

As suggested earlier, amplified spinal cord signals create havoc upstream with devastating effects in sleep architecture. Long-term benzodiazepines cause drug dependence, cognitive dysfunction and alteration in mental health. Short-acting benzodiazepine hypnotic drugs (Ambien, Lunesta) potentiate GABA inhibitory neurotransmitters. Unfortunately, they may cause hallucination in some patients. Medications like Benadryl may work, but the long half-life affect many. Also, these drugs don't help with pain, perhaps except for Amitriptyline.

We have had good response with a new generic drug, Tizanidine, a central muscle relaxant binding not only alpha-2-adrenoreceptors but also imidazole receptors (these may be involved with supraspinal inhibition of spinal reflexes. Many patients report more restful sleep and dream development, but some react negatively with vivid dreams!

Early this next year, Merck & Company plans to launch a new drug that will specifically inhibit orexin, a wake-promoting neurotransmitter present in upper vertebrates in the hypothalamus.

Pain Management

We noted earlier the participation of multiple neurotransmitters in signal augmentation in ascending fibers as well as a descending mechanism of pain control. Many agents have been used off-label with various results such as guaifenesin (Mucinex), originally used by American Indians who obtained the agent from the wood of a specific type of tree. The FDA approved it as an expectorant, later discovering that it inhibited NMDA receptor activity but with mixed results in double-blinded studies in FM.[30.] We all know about the limitations of prostaglandin inhibitors (anti-inflammatory) and potential side effects. The controversy of opioid abuse and efficiency issues go beyond the scope of this book, but we strongly believe in its limited role in central sensitization syndrome.[31]

We also have FDA-approved drugs like pregabalin (Lyrica), with indications for diabetic neuropathy and post-herpetic pain. It binds on the alpha 2 delta subunit protein of voltage-gated calcium channels at the brain and dorsal horn tracts in the spinal cord, reducing $Ca++$ influx. Issues with vasodilation and water retention may affect some.

Milnacipran (Savella), a selective serotonin and norepinephrine reuptake inhibitor, like duloxetine (Cymbalta), may show efficacy in a significant percent of patients. (In most, efficacy reaches 35 percent of the population). These drugs seem to work in descending pathways of pain; side effects vary among them.

Lastly, recall the limited but interesting data and results with spinal cord stimulators? We could see in the future Nano-technology applications that will interact and depolarize ascending nerves in the spinothalamic tracts.

Energy and Concentration

Caffeine is the most widely consumed central nervous system stimulant.[32] Methyl xanthine, a purine base, is the main component in coffee. It is an antagonist of adenosine receptors that work to provide energy production as well as regulate arterial blood flow. (Adenosine is also used to stimulate heart during stress tests.) Additionally, caffeine stimulates noradrenaline receptors and dopamine release. Some people are resistant to these effects, but most will develop unwanted side effects at higher, ingested quantities.

Amphetamines have been used for Attention Deficit Hyperactivity Disorder, appetite suppression and illegal recreational use. They activate neurotransmitters in the brain, mostly catecholamine, norepinephrine and dopamine. Too much may lead to muscle break down, impaired cognitive ability and exacerbate anxiety and cardiac disease.

Histamine H3 receptors are the "new" target for cognitive and sleep disorders. The drug modafinil inhibits noradrenaline reuptake, making the neurotransmitter more abundant at the post-synaptic neuron. Provigil (modafinil) and Nuvigil (armodafinil) are used to treat excessive sleepiness, sleep apnea and shift-work disorders. They are FDA-approved for narcolepsy as well.

Histamine-1 (H1) is involved in most cell activities in the skin: its release provokes the itch sensation. Histamine-2 (H2) is involved in gastric acid secretion. Histamine – 3 (H-3) is the most power-ful wakefulness neuronal fiber type of all. By increasing H3, you increase downstream release of norepinephrine (NE) acetyl choline (Ach), serotonin (5-HT) and dopamine (DE) evoking a variety responses.

The paraventricular thalamic (PVT) nuclei plays an important role in wakefulness, attention, arousal and certain autonomic functions.[33] These nuclei, along with the reticular activating system (RAS) are the two main centers of wakefulness in vertebrates.

The PVT receives one of the densest innervation from the neighboring hypothalamus through the medial forebrain bundle. Within the hypothalamus resides the hypothalamic—hypocretin orexin neurons.

The three main areas to consider are:

1) <u>TMN</u> (tuberomammillary nuclei)- "The wake promoting nuclei" rich in H3.
2) <u>Suprachiasmatic nuclei</u> "The Trigger" near the optic nerve crossing and associated with circadian rhythm.
3) <u>VLP</u> (ventrolateral-preoptic area) associated with NREM sleep.
    - So powerful that destruction of the orexin nuclei (immune destruction of about 4,000 cells) leads to cataplexy or narcolepsy. (Intrusion of REM into Wakefulness.)

Modanifil/Armodafinil activate the TMN nuclei by increasing synaptic H-3.

A shelved drug, Bavisant[34] ($C19H31Cl2N3O2$) is a highly selective oral antagonist to the H3 receptors. We recommend application of this drug for patients with FM and fatigue.

Finally, we have more than 12 biologics or small molecules available for rheumatoid arthritis, a condition that affects 1-2 percent of the worldwide population. There are only a handful available for FM, a condition many times more prevalent. Immune-genetics studies have helped in the development of treatments in RA. FM is much more elusive as we are dealing with hard to reach areas of the deep central nervous system. Hopefully, in the near future, we will have treatments that target main areas in this complex illness.

References

1. Nature 511, 421-427(24 July 2013).
2. J. Attention Disorder 16(9):623-630.
3. Wallace DJ. The history of fibromyalgia, Clauw DJ, eds. Fibromyalgia and Other Pain Syndromes: Lippincott W.S. Wilkins; 2005:1-8.
4. Inanici F. History of fibromyalgia: past to present. Pain Headache rep, 2004 Oct; 8(5):369-78.
5. Puhand, St. Mary's Hospital. P. Republic of Korea: Characteristic changes of unmyelinated nerve fibers in skin of patients with Fibromyalgia (Abstract).
6. Seo- Ho Kim et al. Electron microscopy evidence of Schwann cell ballooning in FM patients compared to controls.
7. Rice, Albrecht et al: Fibromyalgia is not all in your head, new research confirms.
8. Neech G. Neuroendocrine and hormonal perturbations and relations to serotonergic system in fibromyalgia patients. Scandinavian J. Rheumatology Supplement: 2000; 113:8:12.
9. Kacletoff, Kosek, evidence of reduced sympatho-adrenal and hypothalamic-pituitary activity during static muscular work in patient with fibromyalgia. (Abstract).
10. Landis CA, Lentz MJ, et al. Decreased nocturnal Levels of Prolactin and Growth hormones in Women with

Fibromyalgia. J. Clin. Endocrinology, Metab., April 1, 2001; 86(4):1672-1678.

11. Moldofsky H Et al. Musculoskeletal symptoms and non-REM sleep disturbance in patients with "fibrositis syndrome" and healthy subjects. Psychosomatic Medicine, Vol. 37, Issue 4: 341-351.

12. Addolorato G et al. A case of marked cerebellar atrophy in a woman with anorexia nervosa and cerebral atrophy and review of the literature. Int. J. Eating Disorder. 1998 Dec; 24(4):443-7. Sapolsky RM. Arch. Geriatric Psychiatry. 200: 57:925-935.

13. Wood PB. Fibromyalgia syndrome: a central role for the hippocampus. Pages 19-26, 2003.

14. Emad Y Et al. Hippocampus dysfunction may explain symptoms of fibromyalgia syndrome. A study with single voxel magnetic resonance spectroscopy. J. Rheum: 2008 July. (35) (7): 1, 242-4.

15. Tennant F. Brain Atrophy with chronic pain.

16. Jurgen L, Jager L, et al. White and gray matter abnormalities in the brain of patients with fibromyalgia. A diffusion-tension and volumetric imaging study. A&R, Vol. 58, No. 12, Dec 2008, pages 3960 – 3969.

17. Camilleri M, Serotonin in the gastrointestinal tract. Curr. Opin. Endocrinol. Diabetes Obes. Feb 2009; 16(1):53-54.

18. Liu Q, Yang Q, et al. Discovery and characterization of novel tryptophan hydroxylase inhibitors that selectively inhibit serotonin synthesis in the gastrointestinal tract. J. Pharm. Exp. Ther. 2008, 25: 47- 55.

19. Hectkemper M et al. Increased urine Catecholamine's and cortisol in women with irritable bowel syndrome. Am. J. Gastroenterology. 1996. May; 91 (5):906-13.

20. Modafinil and EEG measurement for improvement in "cognitive fog" in fibromyalgia patients. Studies performed at Sitrin Clinic, New Hartford, N.Y.

21. Aparihan, et al. J. Neuroscience 2004, 24 (46):10410-10415.

22. (Sundrepen, D. Clarn. Acad. Radiol. 2007.)

23. Russell IJ et al. Cerebrospinal fluid biogenic amine metabolites in fibromyalgia/fibrositis syndrome and rheumatoid arthritis. Jr. of R. 1992; 35:550-6.

24. Schachter EN, Kmocking K. Out the dream of study pain. N. Engl.J.Med. Vol.347, No.5, August 1,2002.

25. Giesecht T Et al. Subgrouping of fibromyalgia patient based on pressure pain thresholds and psychological factors. Arthritis Rheum. 2003; 20. 743875.

26. Kim DH et al. Association of guanosine triphosphate cyclohydroxilation I gene polymorphisms with fibromyalgia syndrome in a Korean population. J. Rheumatology 2013; 3:316.

27. Arnold LM et al. The fibromyalgia family study. A genome-wide linkage scan study. A & R vol. 65, No. 4. April 2013. Pp. 1122-1128.

28. Yunus MB, Masi ET. Juvenile primary fibromyalgia syndrome: a clinical Study of thirty-three patients and matched normal controls. Arthritis and Rheum. 1985; 28: 138-145.

29. Weiss Becker. I. et al. Childhood trauma and diurnal cortisol disruption in fibromyalgia syndrome. Psychoneuroendocinology. 2006 April: 31(3): 312-314.

30. London M: The truths and myths of the use guaifenesin in fibromyalgia. (mrl@psfc.mit.edu).

31. Ngian GS, et al. The use of opioids in fibromyalgia. Int.J. Rheum. Dis._2011, Feb.14(1):6-11.

32. Nehliq A Et al. Caffeine and the central nervous system. Brain Res Brain. Res. Rev. 1992 May-Aug: 17(2)139-10.

33. Huang et al. Journal of Neurophysiology. 95: 1656-1668, 2006.

34. Weisler RH et al. Randomized Clinical Study of H3 receptor antagonist for the treatment of adults with ADHD, CNS drugs, 2012, May1; 26(5)42-34.

www.ingramcontent.com/pod-product-compliance
Lightning Source LLC
Chambersburg PA
CBHW070244290526
45789CB00004B/1763